YOUR KNOWLEDGE HAS VALUE

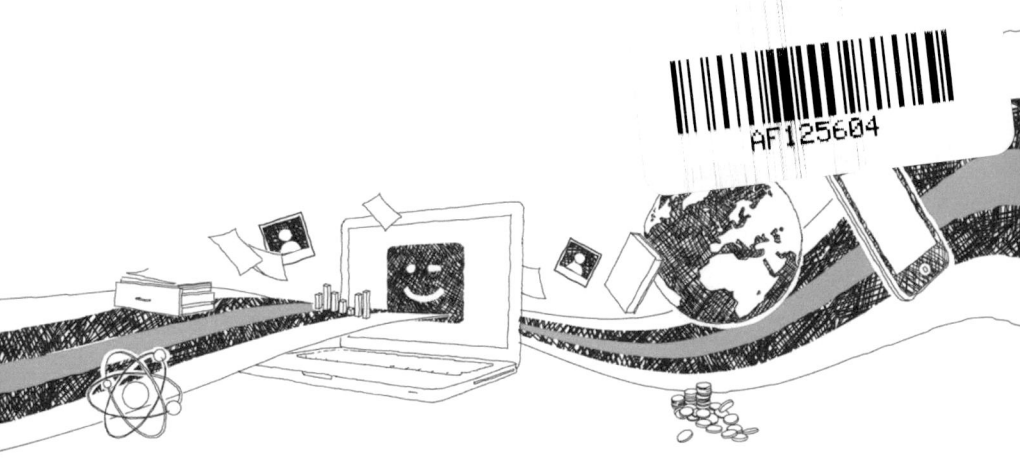
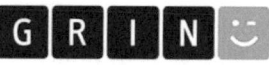

Bibliographic information published by the German National Library:

The German National Library lists this publication in the National Bibliography; detailed bibliographic data are available on the Internet at http://dnb.dnb.de .

Imprint:

Copyright © 2015 GRIN Verlag
Print and binding: Books on Demand GmbH, Norderstedt Germany
ISBN: 9783346116734

This book at GRIN:

https://www.grin.com/document/520401

Jens Nedwal

Aus der Reihe: e-fellows.net schüler-wissen

e-fellows.net (Hrsg.)

Band 2771

The Importance of Structural Integration after Breast Cancer Surgery

GRIN Verlag

GRIN - Your knowledge has value

Since its foundation in 1998, GRIN has specialized in publishing academic texts by students, college teachers and other academics as e-book and printed book. The website www.grin.com is an ideal platform for presenting term papers, final papers, scientific essays, dissertations and specialist books.

Visit us on the internet:

http://www.grin.com/

http://www.facebook.com/grincom

http://www.twitter.com/grin_com

Structural Integration After Breast Cancer Surgery

Jens Nedwal

Jens Nedwal practices structural integration in Wuppertal, Germany. He graduated in 2007 at the Institut für Strukturelle Körpertherapie (Structural Core Therapy Institute) in Nürnberg, Germany. He has worked with oncological patients, particularly post-breast cancer surgery patients, since 2010.

Abstract

Important innovations over the last years have been translated into new breast cancer diagnosis and treatment strategies that are now being integrated into clinical practice. The progress made in imaging diagnostics, primary and reconstructive breast surgery, radiation therapy, and the development of individualized medical treatment strategies has resulted in new tailored and targeted therapies.

The increasing number of new cases per year calls for an analysis of state of the art therapeutic strategies. This article will provide a short view of current breast cancer treatments. It will also discuss the effects of untreated scar tissue, including fascial tension and loss of sensation. In addition, a client example demonstrating the effectiveness of structural integration in cancer aftercare will be presented.

Breast Cancer Background

Basically, there are two major classes of breast cancer: non-infiltrating and infiltrating. The treatment strategies vary based on type.

Non-Infiltrating Tumors

Non-infiltrating epithelial tumors are also known as carcinoma in situ, abbreviated as DCIS (ductal carcinoma in situ). Most cases of breast cancer start in the surface cells (epithels) of the ducts, sometimes in the lobules themselves. As long as the breast cancer is confined to the territory of a lobule, it is called a carcinoma in situ and considered early stage, in which state it can remain for years. In this stage, the disease can be cured by almost 90 percent by surgical removal of the tumor, possibly supplemented by radiation therapy (Goodwin, Parker, Ghersi & Wilcken, 2013). In individual cases, a hormone therapy is applied. Chemotherapy, however, is usually not necessary (Thill & Solomayer, 2014). An unknown percentage of these precursors never develop to invasive breast cancer.

Every fifth woman who receives an initial breast cancer diagnosis has a DCIS (Thill & Solomayer, 2014). So far there are no medical ways to predict which DCIS cancers will later become malignant. Because of this, it is recommended that all women with DCIS seek treatment—even though that may mean unnecessary treatment for some women.

Infiltrating Tumors

There is the large class of so-called infiltrating epithelial tumors, which in turn are divided into different types. These tumors have broken the cell wall of the lobules and grow with very different speed, depending on the cell type, into the surrounding fat tissue of the breast.

Malignant tumors often grow quickly and penetrate aggressively into the surrounding tissue. This penetration is called infiltration or invasion. In addition to being infiltrative, malignant tumors can be destructive, which means they destroy the surrounding tissue. In contrast to benign tumors, malignant tumors usually have no capsule or an incomplete capsule. Malignant tumors often spread along nerves or in lymphatic and blood vessels.

The tumor cells can penetrate into the vessels and be carried away by the blood stream into other parts of the body. They can travel from the blood vessels into the tissue, multiply there, and grow into another tumor. These secondary tumors are called metastases (Kreipe & Friedrichs, 2014).

Treatment

When the diagnosis has shown that breast cancer is present, surgery is necessary in most cases (Kühn & Kümmel, 2014). For decades, surgical removal of the breast was the standard treatment for breast cancer worldwide; the surgeon typically removed the entire breast (radical mastectomy). In addition to the breast tissue and muscles, the lymph nodes of the armpit were removed. Today, gentler surgical alternatives, called breast-conserving surgeries, are available.

Chemotherapy

Adjuvant chemotherapy is a continuation of the surgery, where cytostatic drugs attack the cancer cells—and normal tissue. The cytotoxins affect the cell division process in a very special way; they stop the growth of the cells or prevent further proliferation (Bischoff & Janni, 2014). In special cases, chemotherapy before surgery (neo-adjuventive chemotherapy) can be useful.

Chemotherapy reduces tumor size. It can help to make even bigger breast tumors smaller, so a radical mastectomy is not necessary (Bischoff & Janni, 2014). Although chemotherapy delays the date for the surgery, it does not worsen the prognosis.

Side effects of chemotherapy

Despite careful dosing, chemotherapeutic drugs also affect healthy cells, although to a lesser extent. Low blood cell counts, nausea, vomiting, hair loss, heart damage, kidney damage, and liver damage can occur (Bischoff & Janni, 2014). There are still no clinical studies that consider the effect of chemotherapy on the fascial system.

Radiation

The goal of treatment with ionizing radiation is to destroy possible residual tumor cells or small metastases in the surgical site or in the lymph nodes (Souchon & Friedrichs, 2013). Ionizing radiation attacks the nucleus of the cell. The DNA may be so damaged by the radiation exposure that the cells can no longer divide and multiply. Radiotherapy is always needed if the tumor tissue could not be completely removed and in breast-conserving therapy.

Irradiation of the operated breast is considered essential and is now used more often, because of the increasing use of breast-conserving surgery in recent years. Adjuvant radiation therapy is used to prevent a local recurrence in the immediate area of the operated breast. In general, the radiation starts about three weeks after the surgery, depending on how well the surgical wounds have healed. Irradiation of the breast and lymph nodes takes about six weeks to complete (Souchon & Friedrichs, 2013).

Skin reactions

Skin reactions from radiation include redness, dryness, and underlying immovable fascial tissue. Occasionally, radiation can also lead to an increased pigmentation of the exposed areas of the skin. I found that the irradiated tissue is sensitive to mechanical stimuli and requires caution in terms of sliding and gliding during structural treatment.

Hormone therapy

Scientists have proven that most tumors of the female breast are estrogen-dependent, meaning that the regulation of the growth in these tumors can be influenced by hormones and anti-hormones (Mundhenke & Schütz, 2014). In other words, if you change the hormonal balance of the woman in a very specific way, there is a chance to prevent the development of metastases or a return of the disease (remission).

Forms of hormone therapy for breast cancer.

1   Previously, the ovaries were surgically removed (ovarectomy). Today, there are drugs to turn off ovary function, called *gonadropin-releasing-hormones*. These drugs regulate estrogen production in the ovaries.

2   Certain tumor cells have receptors that register the preference for estrogen. Anti-estrogens and other medications (so called *estrogenrecepting downregulators*) block these receptors so the tumor cell is no longer stimulated to grow.

3   An enzyme (*aromatase*) causes the endogenous formation of estrogens, particularly in fat tissue and in the ovaries. After the onset of menopause, fat tissue is the main endogenous source of estrogen. Aromatase inibitors block the enzyme and the body's production of estrogen.

4   Progesterone, a hormone produced in the ovaries, helps to decrease the blood estrogen

level and additionally inhibits the function of the estrogen receptors.

Fascial reactions

Studies have shown a correlation between high levels of estrogen and high levels of collagen synthesis (Hansen et al., 2008; Talwar, Wong, Svoboda, & Harper, 2006; Claasen et al., 2010). In cases of lower estrogen levels, fascial tension increases over the whole body, especially in scarred areas (Hansen et al., 2008).

Surgical Techniques

Breast-Conserving Surgical Techniques

Through targeted screening measures, breast cancer is increasingly found in early stages when tumors are small. Therefore, breast-conserving surgery is now considered standard treatment for breast cancer. The chances of recovery are just as good, if the tumor is removed with an adequate safety margin and the breast is irradiated afterwards.

A breast-conserving technique is usually possible when a single or multiple small tumors are located in the same quadrant of the breast. Breast-conserving surgery may also be possible for women with large tumors. In some cases, preoperative chemotherapy (neoadjuvant therapy) can shrink the cancer so that the surgeon does not have to amputate the entire breast.

Before the operation, a sentinel lymph node (SLN) is marked with a special process and removed during surgery. During this procedure, the SLN is studied under a microscope to see if cancer cells have spread to the lymph nodes of the armpit. If this is the case, more lymph nodes are removed.

There are three different types of breast-conserving surgical techniques:

1 Only the cancer itself is removed (Lumpectomy)

2 The cancer is removed together with a certain segment of the breast (Segmentectomy)

3 The cancer is removed together with a quadrant of the breast (Quadrantectomy)

By default, radiotherapy is part of a breast-conserving therapy (Witte, 2012).

Modified Radical Mastectomy

A modified radical mastectomy is performed when a breast-preserving approach is not possible because of tumor expansion and the resulting risk of recurrence. Skin-saving forms of mastectomy have not been compared to traditional mastectomy in prospective randomized trials, but in long-term studies and meta-analyses show comparable recurrence rates (Kühn & Kümmel, 2014). The entire mammary tissue, the skin and the nipple-areola-complex and the pectoralis fascia will be removed. The pectoralis musculature is usually maintained. The incision should take into account later reconstruction options.

Reconstruction

After a mastectomy, there are two main types of breast reconstructions: TRAM-flaps or DIEP-flaps.

TRAM-Flaps

TRAM stands for transverse rectus abdominis myocutaneous. In this procedure, a section of the lower abdominal skin, fat, and muscle are used to reconstruct the breast.

This is the most commonly performed type of flap reconstruction (Bassiouny, Maamoun, El-Shasly & Youssef, 2005). One reason is because the lower abdominal tissue has similar qualities to breast tissue and is therefore a good substitute. This procedure has been performed for decades and many surgeons know how to do it. However, the downside of TRAM flaps is that they do cut through muscle, while other types of flap reconstruction avoid this and are therefore "gentler" operations. There are two main types of TRAM flaps:

> • *Free TRAM flap*: In a free TRAM flap, fat, skin, blood vessels, and muscle are cut from the wall of the lower belly and moved up to the chest to rebuild the breast. There is also what's called a "muscle-sparing" free TRAM flap. This means that the surgeon tries to use only part of the rectus abdominis muscle for the flap instead of a large portion of the muscle. Women may recover more quickly and have a lower risk of losing abdominal muscle strength than if they had the full width of muscle taken.

> • *Pedicled (or attached) TRAM flap*: In a pedicled TRAM flap, fat, skin, blood vessels, and muscle from the lower belly wall are moved under the skin up to the chest to rebuild the breast. The blood vessels (artery and vein) of the flap are left attached to their original blood supply in the abdomen. Pedicled TRAM flaps almost always use a large portion of the rectus abdominis muscle and are known as "muscle-transfer" flaps.

> One risk with pedicled TRAM flaps is that the moved tissue may not get enough blood circulation and some of the tissue might die. The blood supply to the pedicled TRAM flap is often less powerful than it is with free flap. With the free flaps, there is also a small risk of the moved tissue not getting enough blood supply—but partial loss of the tissue is much less common.

DIEP Flap

The DIEP (Deep Inferior Epigastric Perforator) flap is the most advanced form of breast reconstruction today (Bruck & Koubenec, 2011). The DIEP procedure uses the patient´s own abdominal skin and fat to reconstruct a natural, warm, soft breast post-mastectomy. Unlike the TRAM flap, the DIEP flap preserves all the abdominal muscles. Only abdominal skin and fat are removed, similar to a "tummy tuck." The skin and fat below the belly button feels very similar to breast tissue.

Sometimes all the lower abdominal tissue is needed to reconstruct the breast and occasionally this cannot be performed as a single flap. In these cases, the lower abdominal tissue can be transplanted as two separate flaps, which are then reconnected on the chest using microsurgery to create one breast. This technique is known as the *stacked DIEP flap* procedure.

Structural Effects of Breast Cancer Surgery

Generally, structural integration (SI) treatments may be held about five years after breast cancer treatment, to allow time to be certain the disease has not returned. The optimum conditions for successful treatment of fascial tissue are carefully healed scars. In general, patients don't have knowledge of the fascial restrictions caused by their scars and other treatments. They do, however, arrive with complaints that are often times a result of these restrictions, which typically include:

- Missing sensation in the operated area and also in the extremities. Stereotypic paresthesia is often exhibited in women with a breast cancer surgery, especially people with breast reconstruction.

- Lymphatic problems, including swelling in the arms.

- Posture changes evident in the thorax, shoulders, and arms. These structural changes may lead to repetitive strain injuries or cumulative trauma disorders, such as epicondylitis or nerve irritation from immobile connective tissue.

- Visceral problems may also stem from postural changes.

Such sequelae [conditions resulting from a prior disease] are usually not considered, by patients, as a result of the surgery, especially if performed years ago; they are often viewed as insignificant. SI practitioners are aware that detecting the patterns created from the incision and reducing the myofascial tension in the affected areas can help to restore more normal functions.

Effect on Arm Patterns

Looking at the breast cancer surgery incision/scar, it is clear that the structures of the Deep and Superficial Front Arm Lines are usually severed. This creates an excessive degree of tension in the deep and superficial back arm lines. In combination, this results in a stronger kyphosis.

In most cases the greatest scarring is present in the area of pectoralis major. The pectoralis minor and its fascia are usually preserved. There is no stereotypical pattern, as there are sometimes several types of incisions during surgery.

Effects on the Abdominal Wall

In TRAM Flap surgery the superficial and deep front lines are significantly distorted, with deep tensions in the fascial network of the abdominal wall. The abdominal muscles insert directly into the thoracolumbar fascia. Contraction of the transversus abdominis tensions the thoracolumbar fascia and pulls it mostly in an anterior direction. Through this connection, the transversus abdominis and the multifidi work collectively to create spinal support.

Structural Integration Post-Breast Cancer Surgery

The treatment of breast cancer scars and adhesions cannot be described as a set modality. Treatment could rather be defined as a "management strategy" aimed at improving tissue quality and mobility. Although the concrete benefits of manual techniques on scars are hard to document, reported benefits include improved skin quality, relieved sensitivity, increased cutaneous hydration, improved scar quality, and better acceptance of the lesion by the patient (Roques, 2002). The management protocols must be flexible enough to promptly recognize complications and risks in order to adjust the timing and application of therapeutic intervention.

The breast is a glandular structure of the superficial fascia layer, separated from the deep fascia of pectoralis major by the retromammary space. It is not supported by muscles, so the fascial membranes take all the stresses of gravity and body movement. Furthermore, the breast does not have usable planes of dissection, so surgical cuts are made bluntly through the tissue. As a result, there can be a great tendency for puckering and pulling as the scar dehydrates and contrasts within its tissue host. There can also be a great tendency of adhesion to the underlying pectoralis major muscle. The scar commonly matted fiber texture.

Treatment of the Scar

The aim of scar management on the mastectomy site is the same as for other body parts— reduction and control of edema and the re-orientation of collagen fibers within the scar. Treatment of scar tissue and adhesions should be aimed first at the breast tissue itself, and secondly at movement between breast and chest wall. A less aggressive approach is advised to limit stress on supporting fascial membranes. The manual techniques I use on the scars have no prescribed style or sequence, but are based on the following principles:

- The goal of the treatment is to loosen the collagen fiber linkages that have developed within the scar and the adhesions between it and the surrounding tissues.

- Effective treatment applies direct pressure to the specific points and directions of resistance. The therapist's finger or hand should not glide over the scar's surface. No, or very little, lubrication should therefore be used.

- Caution is taken on irradiated tissues, which have a very delicate skin and are able to break.

Integration of the Arm Lines

Due to the presence of scar tissue, forces are exerted unevenly through the neck and shoulder girdle. Therefore, after freeing the scar tissue and surrounding areas, I work to faciliate integration of the arm lines and erection of the thorax.

It is common to find significant adhesions and tension in the area of the sternum. Treatment of this area is key as it gives the entire upper torso more space and results in easier breathing and improved head position. I also find it important to clear the clavipectoral fascia in depth. This fascia involves both the pectoralis major and minor and the subclavius muscles and has connections to the neurovascular bundle and lymphoid tissue in this region. It is relatively difficult to find the pectoralis minor and the clavipectoral fascia and to treat it isolated from the pectoralis major (Myers, 2001).

Despite the seemingly clear symmetry, the fascial arm lines have more intersecting links than the corresponding lines in the legs (Myers, 2001). The Deep Front Arm Line (DFAL) begins with the pectoralis minor in the anterior part of the third, fourth and fifth rib. It is advantageous to treat the proximal portions of the DFAL first and then work in the distal parts. I often elongate along the DFAL and the Deep Back Arm Lines to ensure further length of the fascial network of the arm. Due to the large number of intersecting muscles in the arm, it is important to pay attention to the structures that cross the epicondyles and the wrist.

When I work with post-breast cancer surgery clients, I examine the possible connections of fascial tension maintained by their surgery scars. I assess fascial tightness in the deep arm patterns and the thoracolumbar fascia. I try to identify the relationship between specific types of scars and the resulting fascial tension sequelae. I use the following principles when addressing the structural patterns:

1. Treatment is directed at the mechanical restriction identified through evaluation.

2. The goal is to move the tissue barrier towards a normal end-feel and amplitude.

3. Treatment is approached in a layered fashion from superficial to deep, clearing one layer or compartment of restriction before moving to a deeper layer.

4. Gentle touch grading is used during the early stages.

Client Example

As an example, I will describe the treatment for one of my clients, who was 52-years old. Shortly after the initial diagnosis, via ultrasound, the affected lymph nodes were removed. The detected tumor was centered on the left breast muscle. Chemotherapy and radiotherapy were applied before a modified radical mastectomy. The patient decided against a reconstruction of the breast.

Even four to six weeks after surgery, high tension around the sternum remained along the incisions in the pectoralis fascia. A fascial compartment formed and filled with blood and lymph in the area of the sternum. This compartment was punctured five times. In addition, tension in the area of the left elbow and hand arose, which were diagnosed as epicondylitis and tendinitis.

Procedure

I conducted functional analysis and analyzed possible treatment strategies. Each session was conducted once a week for 60 minutes at the same time each week. Session data was collected every other day.

To relieve the tightness in the chest described by the patient, the superfascial layers of the thorax were freed with the goal of increasing pliability. Since latissimus dorsi and teres major belong to the same fascial layer as the pectoralis major through the Superficial Front Arm Line, I found it appropriate to liberate the thorax in a lateral position. This session established a sense of the vertical direction releasing the torso, diaphragm, and hips to allow full expression of the breath.

Following is a list of the sessions with their goals and treatment.

Sessions 1-2: Treated the scar tissue

Loosened and relaxed the superficial and deep scar tissue

Sessions 3-4: Worked on the arm lines and the shoulder girdle

Began systematic liberation of the arm lines from proximal to distal. Improved arm extension. Related connections between the front and the back of the arms.

Sessions 5-6: Freed the thoracal system

Worked on the sides of the pelvis up to the shoulder, creating a lateral centerline and enlargement of the lateral hull. Improved breathing in the lateral center line.

Sessions 7-8: Connected shoulder girdle and the neck

Worked at the deep neck muscles and related to the lungs with the clavicle, upper ribs, and shoulder girdle. Improved verticality of the cervical spine.

Sessions 9-10: Integrated the neck and arm lines into the body

Oriented the arms to the center line. Created a balance between the waist/neck and neck/head. Horizontalized the head.

Results

One result of the treatment was a reduction of the compartment along the sternum, which was reduced in the first two treatments significantly and prevented another puncture. In general, the head and neck moved into an appropriate line and, as described above, the thorax had been given more space. The left arm was freed from adhesions around the epicondyles.

Through the course of treatment, a deeper and finer sense of the body came to light. The areas where sensation was diminished at the beginning of the sessions were clearly perceived by the ending sessions, and had transformed themselves. Throughout the ten sessions the patient experienced a high frequency of heat, color, and visual sensations and also a finer and deeper experience of the sensations of pain. This suggests that tactile stimulation, especially fascial stimulation, can amplify the patient's sensory refinement.

Discussion

Prior investigations in post-breast cancer surgery treatment often adopted random physical techniques to reduce symptoms without necessarily determining their origin. However, as a structural integration practitioner, I realize that fascial restrictions caused by breast cancer treatment are a determining factor in the sequelae of oncological aftercare.

Rather than isolating these conditions (swelling, loss of range of motion, loss of sensation) and treating them separately, the structural integrator can identify the effects on the fascial network of deeply scarred tissue, and then effectively work on the patient's situation. The preliminary finding of the client example above shows that structural integration reduced such sequelae effectively.

Structural integration, in individual cases, can provide positive physical and sensory consequences and can be used used in cancer aftercare to improve patient function and reduce aberrant discomforts.

Resources

Deutsche Krebsgesellschaft e. V. (The German Cancer Society) www.krebsgesellschaft.de

Informationsseiten der Deutschen Gesellschaft für Senologie (Breast Cancer Studies) www.brustkrebs-studien.de

Robert Koch-Institut, Neue Daten zu Krebs in Deutschland. (The Robert Koch Institute, New Data on Cancer in Germany) http://www.rki.de/DE/Content/Service/Presse/Pressemitteilungen/2013/14_2013.html

References

Bassiouny, M.M., Maamoun, S.I., El-Shazly, S.D., & Youssef, O.Z. (2005). TRAM flap for immediate post mastectomy reconstruction: Comparison between pedicaled and free transfer. *Journal of Egyptian National Cancer Institute*, *17*(4), 231-238.

Bischoff, J. (2014). Chemotherapie mit oder ohne zielgerichtete Substanzen beim metastasierten

Mammakarzinom. *Arbeitsgemeinschaft Gynakologische Onkologie e. V.*

Bruck, J. C., & Koubenec, H. J. (2011). Wiederaufbau der Brust nach Amputation. Retrieved from http://www.brustkrebs-info.de/patienten-info/index.php?datei=patienten-info/brustkrebs-therapie/op_plastische-chirurgie.htm

Claassen, H., Steffen, R., Jassenpflug, J., Varoga, D., Wruck, C. J., . . . Pufe, T. (2010). 17β-estradiol reduces expression of MMP-1, -3, and -13 in human primary articular chondrocytes from female patients cultured in a three dimensional alginate system. *Cell and Tissue Research, 342*(2), 283-293.

Fisher B., Anderson S. Conservative surgery for the management of invasive and noninvasive carcinoma of the breast: NSABP trials. National Surgical Adjuvant Breast and Bowel Project. World J Surg 1994; 18(1):63-69.

Goodwin A., Parker S., Ghersi D., & Wilcken N. (2013). Post-operative radiotherapy for ductal carcinoma in situ of the breast. *Cochrane Database of Systematic Reviews.* Nov 21; 11:CD000563.

Hansen, M., Koskinen, S. O., Petersen, S. G., Doessing, S., Frystyk, J., . . . Langberg, H. (2008). Ethinyl oestradiol administration in women suppresses synthesis of collagen in tendon in response to exercise. *Journal of Physiology, 586*(12), 3005-3016.

Kreipe, H. H. & Friedrichs, K. (2014). Pathologie. *Arbeitsgemeinschaft Gynakologische Onkologie e. V.*

Kühn, T. & Kümmel, S. (2014). Operative Therapie des Mammakarzinoms unter onkologischen Aspekten. *Arbeitsgemeinschaft Gynakologische Onkologie e. V.*

Myers, T. (2001). *Anatomy trains: Myofascial meridians for manual and movement therapists.* Elsevier: Churchill Livingstone.

Mundhenke, U. & Schütz, F. Antihormonelle und zielgerichtete Therapie des metastasierten Mammakarzinoms. *Arbeitsgemeinschaft Gynakologische Onkologie e. V.*

NZGG. New Zealand Guidelines Group: Management of early breast cancer. Wellington: 2009

Roques, C. (2002). Massage applied to scars. *Wound Repair and Regeneration*, 10(2), 126-128.

Souchon, R. & Friedrichs, K. (2013). Strahlentherapie. *Arbeitsgemeinschaft Gynakologische Onkologie e. V.*

Talwar, R. M., Wong, B. S., Svoboda, K., & Harper, R. P. (2006). Effects of estrogen on chondrocyte proliferation adn collagen synthesis in skeletally mature articular cartilage. *Journal of Oral and Maxillofacial Surgery, 64*(4), 600-609.

Thill, M. & Solomayer, E. F. (2014). Diagnostik und Therapie primärer und metastasierter Mammakarzinome. *Arbeitsgemeinschaft Gynakologische Onkologie e. V.* Retrieved from www.ago-online.de

Voogd A. C., Nielsen M. Peterse J.L., Blichert-Toft M., Bartelink H., Overgaard M., van Tienhoven G., Andersen K.W., Sylvester R.J., van Dongen J. A. Differences in risk factors for local and distant recurrence after breast-conserving therapy or mastectomy for stage I and II breast cancer: pooled results of two large European randomized trials. J. Clin Oncol 2001; 19(6): 1688-1697

Witte, F. (2012). Leitlinie für die Diagnostik, Therapie und Nachsorge des Mammakarzinoms. *Aktualisierung Krebsinformationsdienst des Deutschen Krebsforschungszentrums.*

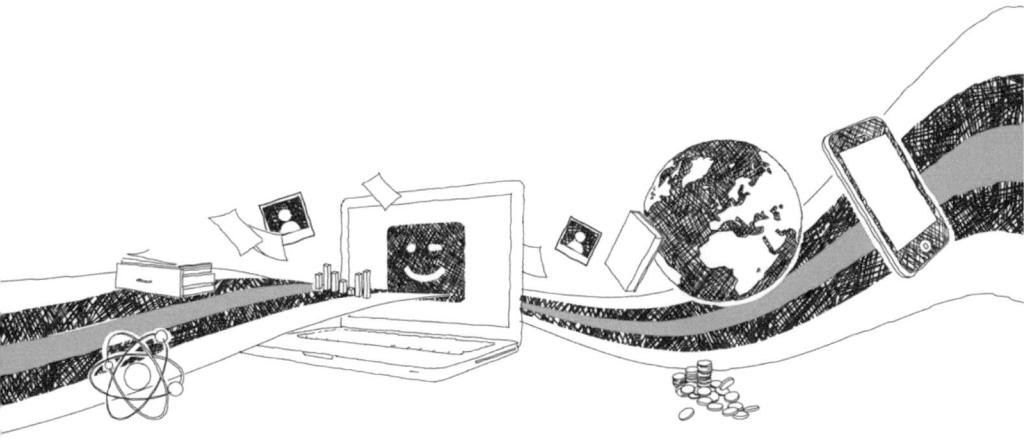
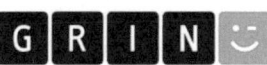